Medical Collaboration
for
Nutritional Therapists

Lucille Leader

Foreword by Professor Leslie Findley
& Dr Serena Leader

Edited by Dr Geoffrey Leader

DENOR PRESS

ISBN 978 0 9526056 5 2

British Library Cataloguing in Publication Data. A catalogue record for this book is available from the British Library.

Published by Denor Press Ltd
PO Box 12913 London N12 8ZR
www.denorpress.com

Cover Design by Commecial Campaigns from an idea by Geoffrey Leader
Layout and Design by Commecial Campaigns: www.commercialcampaigns.com

Printed by: Lightning Source, Milton Keynes, UK

Lucille Leader Dip ION MBANT
email: denor@dial.pipex.com

Lecturer in Nutritional Therapy at Westminster University,
School of Integrated Health, London, UK

Nutrition Director, The London Pain Relief and Nutritional Support Clinic,
The Highgate Hospital, London, UK

Council Member, Food and Health Forum, Royal Society of Medicine, London, UK

Member of the British Society for Ecological Medicine, London, UK

*Lectured in Europe for The European Parkinson's Disease Association (EPDA)
in Specialised Nutritional Management in Parkinson's Disease, in the USA for
the Parkinson's Resource Organisation (Meeting of the Minds), in Vienna at
the first Congress for Sexuality and Nutrition in Parkinson's Disease, in South
Africa for the Johannesburg Parkinson's Disease Society and at UK
Parkinson's Disease Societies. She has received a "Quality of Life in
Parkinson's Award" in the USA and the CAM "Highly Commended
Outstanding Practice Certificate Award" in the UK.
Amongst other publications as author, Lucille Leader is
co-author of five successful books on Parkinson's Disease.*

Geoffrey Leader MB ChB FRCA
email: denor@dial.pipex.com

Medical Director, The London Pain Relief and Nutritional Support Clinic,
The Highgate Hospital, London, UK

Consultant Anaesthetist, The Highgate Hospital, London, UK
The Wellington Hospital, London, UK

Formerly Chairman of the Anaesthetic Department,
Senior Anaesthetic Consultant, Senior Lecturer, Pain Clinic Consultant,
Director of Intensive Care Unit, Newham General Hospital
(The London Hospital Medical College, London University, UK)

*Lectured in Europe for The European Parkinson's Disease Association (EPDA)
in Specialised Nutritional Management in Parkinson's Disease, in the USA for
the Parkinson's Resource Organisation (Meeting of the Minds), in Vienna at
the first Congress for Sexuality and Nutrition in Parkinson's Disease, in South
Africa for the Johannesburg Parkinson's Disease Society and at UK
Parkinson's Disease Societies. He has received a "Quality of Life in
Parkinson's Award" in the USA. Geoffrey Leader is the co-author of
four successful books on Parkinson's Disease.
He has contributed to peer-reviewed anaesthetic journals and is especially
interested in the nutritional support of patients with acute and chronic illness.*

i

Dr Serena Leader MB BS BSc DRCOG MRCP MRCGP

*Dr Serena Leader has always championed a multidisciplinary approach
to healthcare which includes nutrition.
She has an appreciation of the pivotal role of the General Practitioner (GP)
in coordinating multidisciplinary care.*

*Her medical background has been in hospital medicine, including posts in
London at The Royal Free Hospital, The Hammersmith Hospital
and The Brompton Hospital.*

*She has obtained Memberships of both the Royal College of Physicians
and The Royal College of General Practitioners in London, UK.
She practices as a GP in London.*

Professor Leslie Findley KLCJ TD MD FRCP FACP
email: ljfindley@uk-consultants.co.uk

Professor of Health Sciences (Neurology) at South Bank University, London, UK.
Senior Consultant Neurologist at the Essex Neurosciences Unit, Oldchurch
Hospital, Romford, Essex, UK.

*Professor Findley is Founder and Chairman of the National Tremor Foundation
and a Trustee of the National ME Centre for Fatigue Syndromes.
He is a member of the Medical Advisory Panel of the European Parkinson's
Disease Association (EPDA.), member of the WHO Working Party
on Parkinson's Disease and past Chairman of The Parkinson's Disease Society
of the United Kingdom.*

*He is a promoter of the multi-disciplinary approach, which includes nutrition,
to the management of Parkinson's Disease and other neurological illness.*

*He has written the Foreword to the well-acclaimed book on the subject of this
integrated approach, "Parkinson's Disease - The Way Forward!"
(Denor Press: ISBN 0 9526056 8 6) together with
Dr Geoffrey Leader, Lucille Leader, Professor Aroldo Rossi,
Dr Lia Rossi-Prosperi and other eminent specialists
in the field of Parkinson's Disease.
He is also the author of the Foreword in the successful book
"Parkinson's Disease - Reducing Symptoms with Nutrition and Drugs"
(Denor Press: ISBN 978 0 9526056 4 5)
by Lucille Leader and Dr Geoffrey Leader
His main clinical and research interests are movement disorders
and fatigue syndromes.*

Foreword
Message from the General Practitioner

I must congratulate the author of this book for setting gold standards
of practice in the world of nutritional therapy.

Delivering a high standard of care depends very much on excellent
communication by the nutritional therapist, not only with patients and their
carers, but also with the main health professionals responsible for their care.

The General Practitioner (GP) is often the first port of call when a patient
presents with clinical symptoms and is therefore responsible for making the
first clinical assessment. After taking a thorough history and examination
of the patient, a working diagnosis may be established and a suitable
management plan devised incorporating appropriate investigations and
subsequent treatment. It may be necessary to refer the patient to other
healthcare professionals including hospital consultants, physiotherapists,
dieticians, counsellors, social and occupational services.

The GP is the patient's prime advocate and orchestrates all aspects of his
or her care.

At the present time, there are no formal referral pathways to refer patients
to private nutritional therapists. Patients are responsible for choosing their
own fully accredited nutritional therapist and keeping their GP informed.

It is advisable that with the patient's consent, the clinical nutritionist writes
to the GP with a request to share medical information. In the interest of safe
management, it would be important for the nutritional therapist to be fully
informed directly by the medical practitioner, of the working diagnosis,
results of relevant investigations and treatment plan to date, as well as the
patient's past medical history and all current medication.

Careful consideration must be given to ensure that the proposed nutritional
management plan is fully compatible with the patient's medical history. This
must include an assessment of possible adverse drug-nutrient interactions.

Clinical nutritionists must work only within their clinical boundaries and
must at the earliest recognition of diagnostic dilemmas or limitations within

their clinical remit, refer the patient back to their General Practitioner or Specialist as a matter of urgency.

The GP must be alerted of any unexplained findings during investigation and assessment by the clinical nutritionist.

Clinical nutritionists can be of great support in the management of patients, but must work in close collaboration with the medical team responsible for the patient's care.

Dr Serena Leader MB BS BSc DRCOG MRCP MRCGP
General Practitioner
London, UK

Foreword
From the Desk of the Consultant Neurologist

In the last decades, in order to provide the optimal care that is the most effective for our patients, medical management of disease has become increasingly multi-disciplinary.

In my own area, neurology, we have not yet explained the process of premature cellular dysfunction/death, which is underlying in most neurodegenerative disorders, such as Parkinson's disease. In this, and most other areas of medicine, the physician has become highly reliant on the nutritionist and other experts, to ensure that the individual patient has a nutritional programme, which will lend itself to the preservation of health of the whole person, and maximise the potential for cellular survival. Thus, good understanding, and communication between members of the multi-disciplinary team, such as the nutritionist and physician, is absolutely essential if best care is to be offered to our patients.

With these thoughts in mind, Lucille Leader, one of our leading nutritionists, has produced this small practical volume, which defines the "collaboration and communication" process for members of the multi-disciplinary team, with specific emphasis on the nutritionist. This book provides precise guidelines as to the transfer of information between the members of the multi-disciplinary team, accepting that the general practitioner/medical specialist, is the lead, or conductor, of the "therapeutic orchestra".

This volume is original in concept and content. It is of practical importance. Whilst aimed as a guide to the nutritionist, I am sure that my medical colleagues would benefit from reading it, as whilst we, as physicians, play important roles within the multi-disciplinary team, some of us need reminding that as part of a team, we are a more effective as medical practitioners.

In essence, the team is only as good as its weakest player – I think the ideas in this volume will make us all stronger players.

Professor Leslie J Findley KLCJ TD MD FRCP FACP
Consultant Neurologist
London, UK

From the Office of the Editor

As a consultant anaesthetist, I work within the framework of a multidisciplinary team which is responsible for the care of chronically ill patients. I am acutely aware of how nutritional support underpins the various disciplines and may vitally affect outcome.

It is therefore essential for myself, as well as the General Practitioner (GP) and other medical colleagues, to remain in close contact, not only with the team as a whole, but especially with the nutritional therapist.

This is in order to exchange medical information which may be pertinent to the management of the patient. Of particular concern is the avoidance of drug-nutrient interactions and the peri-operative planning of drugs and nutritional support for any surgery.

During the many years that I have worked with the author, I have noted that her dynamic contact with the medical profession has resulted in recognition of the potential benefit of biochemically based nutritional support in patient management.

Dr Geoffrey Leader MB ChB FRCA
Consultant Anaesthetist
London, UK

Dedication

To my Colleagues

Introduction
By the Clinical Nutritionist

When I was a student, a recently-qualified nutritional therapy graduate was threatened with court action by a patient's General Practitioner (GP). This was because the health of the patient had deteriorated.

On questioning by the GP, it emerged that the patient had attended a nutritional therapy clinic and had been prescribed various nutritional supplements and a specialised diet. The GP, not understanding the reason for the nutritional recommendations, assumed that these had been responsible for destabilising the patient. Fortunately, in this case, the nutritional therapist was able to justify her recommendations.

Since qualifying, I have never given nutritional advice without first obtaining relevant details from the GP. In my clinical experience, clients/patients are sometimes reluctant to divulge all of their medical history. Furthermore, there are occasions when a GP deliberately does not disclose certain facts to a patient but would consider it important to communicate this information to the therapist.

With the patient's consent, it is essential that there is exchange of information between the GP and nutritional therapist. It ensures doing one's best to fully understand all aspects of a case before giving advice. This is an essential part of good clinical practice.

I have compiled this book in response to the many requests I have received from colleagues and students. It is my sincere hope that my recommendations will serve as a helpful guide.

Lucille Leader Dip ION MBANT
Nutritional Therapist
London, UK

Medical Collaboration
for
Nutritional Therapists

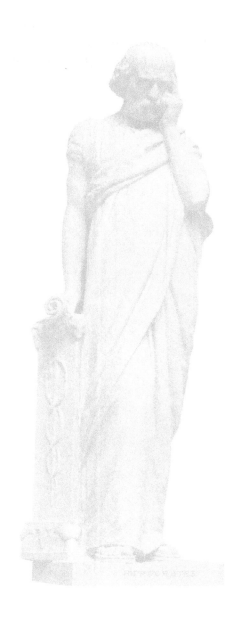

Disclaimer

The recommendations presented in this book are the personal protocols of the author. They definitely are not intended to replace the personal method of practice or initiative of any clinical nutritionist.

This text should be considered merely as a guide to the concept of responsible practice - in the interests of patient safety.

As such, the author, editor and contributors to this manuscript cannot accept responsibility for any problems arising from the application of any of the recommendations contained therein.

Contents

1

Q. What is Collaborative Medicine?

*A. Collaborative Medicine is the interface
between the nutritional practitioner
and the existing healthcare team.*

This includes:

- general practitioner (GP), who is the coordinator of the patient's healthcare team
- relevant medical specialist, including neurologists, gastroenterologists, dermatologists, surgeons etc.
- speech therapist
- occupational therapist
- physiotherapist
- nutritional therapist/dietician
- psychologist/psychiatrist
- other health professionals
- care givers (carers)

Notes:

Q. What is the Importance of Integrated Collaboration?

A. *Collaboration between the nutritional therapist and the medical practitioner provides exchange of information*

For:

- *optimum and comprehensive assessment* of patient health status

- *patient safety and continuity of care* (mutual links established)

- *assistance* - ability to request further information, additional referrals, biochemical tests

- *nutritional care plan* - provides recommendations

- *legal* implications – the clinical nutritionist may need to be able to defend a protocol offered to a patient and the fact that the patient's medical practitioner is aware of the nutritional input can be protective

Notes:

The Initial Approach (Two Options)

Option 1. The prospective patient requests a letter with relevant details about his/her health status from the General Practitioner (GP). This should be sent/given to the clinical nutritionist/nutritional therapist.
(See pages 9-17)

Option 2. The clinical nutritionist/nutritional therapist requests a letter from the GP with relevant details about the health status of the prospective client/patient.
(See page 19)

Notes:

Option 1

1. After initial contact by a patient, explain that you prefer to work in collaboration with patients' General Practitioners (GPs) as this is in the best and safe interests of patients.

2. Arrange to send him/her information about your clinic which can be discussed with the GP. Add that should the GP wish to speak to you about your work, your telephone number is listed on the information you are providing.

The Information Pack

This contains:

- the relevant general nutritional approach of your clinic to the patient's individual pathology

- the request for a GP letter with information about the case and acknowledgement that the client/patient has requested "nutritional assessment and recommendation"

Notes:

Information for the General Practitioner

Lucille Leader Dip ION MBANT
Nutritional Therapist

Highgate Hospital
View Road
London N6 4DJ

Tel: 020 84454550
Fax: 020 84464504
Email: denor@dial.pipex.com

Information for Multiple Sclerosis Patients
This clinic works exclusively in co-operation with patients' existing healthcare teams. A letter with relevant information about your medical history should be obtained from the General Practitioner (GP). It should also acknowledge your request for "Nutritional Assessment and Recommendation".

Your GP should address the referral to: Lucille Leader Dip ION MBANT
The Highgate Hospital
View Road
London
N6 4DJ

Kindly ensure that your GP includes any recent tests or radiology results. This clinic informs GPs of nutritional assessments and recommendations.

Specialised Nutritional Management
Specialised nutritional support is based on the biochemical individuality of each patient. The cellular status of each patient, established by medical laboratory tests, dictates the nutritional recommendations and management. Cellular environment may need to be up/down-regulated according to test results.

Routine medical, as well as specialized biochemical tests for nutritional status of cells (vitamins, minerals, essential fatty acids), digestive enzymes, intestinal permeability, allergy, and comprehensive stool analyses are performed by accredited medical laboratories, when indicated.

Cell membrane support is essential in neurological degenerative disease. Deficiencies of essential fatty acids as well as nutrients which affect general metabolism and oxidative stress are addressed.

Regulation of digestive enzymes, gut membrane integrity and bowel function is addressed.

Diet is optimized, taking into account those foods which are contraindicated, substituting with nutritious alternatives. Problems are addressed which are associated with difficulty in chewing and dysphagia. Indications for specialised tube feeding are taken into account. Weight control and problems of malabsorption are addressed.

Lucille Leader Dip ION MBANT
Nutritional Therapist

Highgate Hospital
View Road
London N6 4DJ

Tel: 020 84454550
Fax: 020 84464504
Email: denor@dial.pipex.com

Information for Patients requesting Nutritional Assessment and Recommendation

This clinic works exclusively in co-operation with patients' existing healthcare teams. A letter with relevant information about your medical history should be obtained from the General Practitioner (GP). It should also acknowledge your request for "Nutritional Assessment and Recommendation".

Your GP should address the referral to: Lucille Leader Dip ION MBANT
The Highgate Hospital
View Road
London
N6 4DJ

Kindly ensure that your GP includes any recent blood, stool, urine or radiology test results. This clinic informs General Practitioners of nutritional assessments and recommendations.

Aspects of Nutritional Therapy

Biochemical Tests

People with chronic illness tend to demonstrate, on a cellular level, that they have nutritional deficiencies. These could include aspects of cellular energy metabolism (the citric acid cycle), the integrity of cellular membranes, the essential fatty acids, vitamins, minerals and antioxidant enzymes.

Patients undergo routine medical tests if indicated as well as nutritional biochemical tests to assess the nutritional status of cells.

Intestinal Status

Intestinal status is assessed – including digestive enzymes, intestinal permeability, intestinal dysbiosis, occult blood, parasites and other parameters, as indicated. Bowel function is regulated, including management of chronic constipation or diarrhoea (differential diagnosis taken into account).

Diet

Diet recommended is appropriate to the individual pathology presented. Dietary recommendations are given to those patients who take pharmaceutical medication as well as those who do not. Drug-nutrient interactions are taken into consideration when planning the nutritional program.

For those suffering from malabsorption or dysphagia, specialised feeding may be recommended. Cooperation with a Speech Therapist may be indicated if necessary.

For those patients with special needs, sublingual supplements, tube feeding and intravenous nutritional support may be recommended to the General Practitioner.

Nutritional Supplementation
Nutritional supplementation is recommended for patients who demonstrate any cellular nutritional deficiencies, have problems of digestion, absorption or increased intestinal permeability. Supplementation is based on the biochemical individuality of patients.

Lucille Leader Dip ION MBANT
Nutritional Therapist

Highgate Hospital
View Road
London N6 4DJ

Tel: 020 84454550
Fax: 020 84464504
Email: denor@dial.pipex.com

General Information for Parkinson's Disease Patients
This clinic works exclusively in co-operation with patients' existing healthcare teams. A letter with relevant information about your medical history should be obtained from the General Practitioner (GP). It should also acknowledge your request for "Nutritional Assessment and Recommendation".

Your GP should address the referral to: Lucille Leader Dip ION MBANT
The Highgate Hospital
View Road
London
N6 4DJ

Kindly ensure that your GP includes any recent blood, stool, urine or radiology test results. This clinic informs General Practitioners of nutritional assessments and recommendations.

Nutritional Aspects for Parkinson's Disease Patients
Biochemical Tests
People with chronic illness tend to demonstrate, on a cellular level, that they have nutritional deficiencies. These could include aspects of cellular energy metabolism (the citric acid cycle), the integrity of cellular membranes, the essential fatty acids, vitamins, minerals and antioxidant enzymes.

Patients undergo routine medical tests if indicated as well as nutritional biochemical tests to assess the nutritional status of cells.

Intestinal Status
Intestinal status is assessed – including digestive enzymes, intestinal permeability, intestinal dysbiosis, occult blood, parasites and other parameters, as indicated. Bowel function is regulated, including management of chronic constipation or diarrhoea (differential diagnosis taken into account).

Diet
Diet recommended is appropriate to the individual pathology presented. Dietary recommendations are given to those patients who take pharmaceutical

medication as well as those who do not. Drug-nutrient interactions are taken into consideration when planning the nutritional program.

For those suffering from malabsorption or dysphagia, specialised feeding may be recommended. Cooperation with a Speech Therapist may be indicated if necessary.

For those patients with special needs, sublingual supplements, tube feeding and intravenous nutritional support may be recommended to the General Practitioner.

Nutritional Supplementation
Nutritional supplementation is recommended for patients who demonstrate any cellular nutritional deficiencies, have problems of digestion, absorption or increased intestinal permeability. Supplementation is based on the biochemical individuality of patients.

Lucille Leader Dip ION MBANT
Nutritional Therapist

Highgate Hospital
View Road
London N6 4DJ

Tel: 020 84454550
Fax: 020 84464504
Email: denor@dial.pipex.com

General Information for Parkinson's Disease Patients
This clinic works exclusively in co-operation with patients' existing healthcare teams. A letter with relevant information about your medical history should be obtained from the General Practitioner (GP). It should also acknowledge your request for "Nutritional Assessment and Recommendation".

Your GP should address the referral to: Lucille Leader Dip ION MBANT
The Highgate Hospital
View Road
London
N6 4DJ

Kindly ensure that your GP includes any recent blood, stool, urine or radiology test results. This clinic informs General Practitioners of nutritional assessments and recommendations.

Nutritional Aspects for Parkinson's Disease Patients
When to Take Drugs in Relation to Food
Side effects of dopaminergic drugs may often be reduced by an understanding of drug-nutrient interactions.

 In order to optimise the absorption of L-dopa, patients are advised which foods are chemically compatible with absorption of this drug as well as the timing of taking L-dopa in relation to different food groups.

Biochemical Tests
The spectrum of tests recommended covers routine medical tests when indicated (including haematology, biochemistry, ferritin, CRP, thyroid, parasites and other tests). In addition, tests are recommended to establish the nutritional status of cells, to assess intestinal status including digestive enzymes, intestinal permeability and other parameters.

People with Parkinson's Disease, as well as those with other chronic illnesses, tend to demonstrate that they have cellular nutritional deficiencies which may affect metabolism, oxidative stress and other biochemical pathways.

continued over ➡

Nutritional Supplements
Patients who demonstrate any cellular nutritional deficiencies and problems of digestion and absorption, are recommended to the use of appropriate nutritional supplements. In some cases, specialised feeding may be recommended.

Bowel Function
Constipation, is dynamically managed. Causes of diarrhoea and other bowel problems are addressed. The clinic works in association with gastroenterologists, if indicated.

Diet and Weight Control
Specialised dietary recommendations are given to those patients who are on L-dopa medication as well as those who are not.

The General Practitioner (GP), Neurologist and other Health Professionals
The clinic always works in co-operation with the drug regime and recommendations of patients' individual Neurologists and General Practitioners as well as with other members of the multidisciplinary management team.

Option 2

If the person applying for an appointment is not comfortable about requesting a letter from the General Practitioner (GP), ask permission to write to the GP yourself requesting information about the prospective patient. Enclose information about your clinic.

Lucille Leader Dip ION MBANT
Nutritional Therapist

Highgate Hospital
View Road
London N6 4DJ

Tel: 020 84454550
Fax: 020 84464504
Email: denor@dial.pipex.com

8th January 2009

Dr K Smith
The Gell Surgery
3 Hill Crescent
London N5 2JL

Dear Dr Smith

Re: John Rabitt, DOB 12.01.1948, 12 Long Way, East Finchley, N2 6AB

Your patient, Mr Rabitt, has approached me for nutritional assessment and recommendation. He states that he is suffering from Parkinson's Disease.

In the interests of patient safety, I work exclusively in collaboration with the general practitioner of a patient. It would therefore be appreciated by Mr Rabitt if you would be kind enough to send me a letter with relevant details of his health history and acknowledge the patient's request for nutritional assessment and recommendation.

Assuring you of my cooperation with you at all times in the best and safe interests of Mr Rabitt.

Yours sincerely

Lucille Leader Dip ION MBANT
Nutritional Therapist

see over for Patient Confidentiality ➡

Patient Confidentiality

It may be wise to ask the prospective client/patient to send a letter to you, the Nutritional Therapist, giving the General Practitioner (GP) permission to release information to yourself. This can then be included with your letter to the GP which requests clinical information.

Specimen Letter to send to the Prospective Client

This should be signed and returned to you for inclusion with your letter to the GP requesting clinical information (see page 19).

Name: Edwina Moss

Address: 3 Albert Drive, London N12 7EF

Date: 31 September 2009

General Practitioner: Dr Timothy Green

Address: 21 Edgware Gardens, London N12 4JK

Dear Dr Green

I hereby give you my permission to disclose relevant clinical information to Nutritional Therapist ....(your name). This may include the results of any tests and special investigations. I have approached ....(your name) for nutritional assessment and recommendations.

Thank you for your kind attention and cooperation.

Yours faithfully

Signature: ....

Edwina Moss

Biochemical Tests and Where they are Available

The NHS provides the following tests which are helpful baselines for nutritional therapists. The therapist could request the assistance of the GP in obtaining these tests within his or her NHS remit. (See the request letter).

- Haematology, Biochemistry, Ferritin, CRP
- Fasting Lipids
- Fasting Glucose
- Glucose Tolerance and Insulin, Glycosylated Haemoglobin
- Thyroid Profile
- PSA (prostate specific antigen)
- Vitamin B12
- Folate
- Vitamin D3
- Zinc
- Hormone Profile
- Urine (culture and sensitivity)
- Stool Tests for parasites and blood

Private medical, as well as nutritional tests can be carried out by:

- Biolab Medical Unit, London UK (Tel: 020 7636 5959)
- Genova Diagnostics, London UK (Tel: 020 8336 7750)
- The Doctors Laboratory London UK (Tel: 020 7460 4800)
- Neurotech, Bournmouth UK (Tel: 01202 510910)
- Acumen Laboratory, UK (Tel: 07707 877175)
- Other laboratories

Important Note: *The GP name and address must appear on private test request forms (request copies to Nutritional Therapist, with address). Test results will automatically go directly to the GP. If you do not receive copies of the results, telephone the GP practice and ask the secretary to assist by sending these to you, explaining that you had requested them. The patient may also ask for the results to be sent to you.*

Notes:

Initial Correspondence with the General Practitioner (GP)

Biochemical Tests: Request to the NHS Medical Practitioner

If your patient has budgetary constraints, write and ask the GP if it is possible, within his remit, to carry out any necessary tests, which you know are available on the NHS.

Lucille Leader Dip ION MBANT
Nutritional Therapist

Highgate Hospital
View Road
London N6 4DJ

Tel: 020 84454550
Fax: 020 84464504
Email: denor@dial.pipex.com

8th January 2009

Dr K Smith
The Gell Surgery
3 Hill Crescent
London N5 2JL

Dear Dr Smith

Re: Sarah Jones, DOB: 14/01/1945, 136 Highcroft, Glasgow, G4 8FG

Thank you for your kind referral of Mrs Jones for nutritional assessment and recommendation. She presented with Parkinson's Disease diagnosed in May 2000. She also suffers from chronic fatigue, hair loss, dry skin, chronic diarrhoea and intermittently passes blood and mucus in the stool.

Mrs Jones does not have private health insurance. In view of her history, as she has budgetary constraints, it would be appreciated if it could be within your remit to assist her with the following routine medical tests:

1. Full Haematology
2. Full Biochemistry
3. Ferritin
4. Thyroid profile (TSH / T4 / T3, Thyroid Auto-antibodies)
5. CRP
6. Glucose tolerance (insulin and glucose)
7. Parasites (stool specimens)

Other specialised tests for nutritional cellular status will be carried out at a private medical laboratory.

I shall report the results and my recommendations to you.

I am concerned about the abdominal symptoms. I have asked Mrs Jones to make an appointment with you for your kind assessment.

I look forward to co-operating with you in the best interests of Mrs Jones.

Thank you for your kind attention.

Yours sincerely

Lucille Leader Dip ION MBANT
Nutritional Therapist

Medical Response!
This patient was referred to a gastroenterologist and Crohn's Disease was diagnosed. Tests demonstrated hypothyroidism.

Initial Correspondence with the General Practitioner (GP)

Initial Report of Test Results and Recommendations to the GP

Lucille Leader Dip ION MBANT
Nutritional Therapist

Highgate Hospital
View Road
London N6 4DJ

Tel: 020 84454550
Fax: 020 84464504
Email: denor@dial.pipex.com

8th January 2009

Dr K Smith
The Gell Surgery
3 Hill Crescent
London N5 2JL

Dear Dr Smith

Re: Sue Jay, DOB: 14/01/1945, 136 Highcroft, Glasgow, G4 8FG

Thank you for your kind letter with information about the above patient who has requested nutritional assessment and recommendation. She was diagnosed with Parkinson's Disease in March 2000 and is taking L-dopa (*Sinemet-Plus*).

Nutritional Biochemical tests demonstrated the following deficiencies:

Essential Fatty Acids
Omega 6
Omega 3

Mineral Analysis
Zinc
Magnesium

Functional B Vitamins
B1 (borderline)
B2
B3

Biotin

Vitamin B12

continued over ➡

25

Folate
Results pending

Glutathione Peroxidase (selenium dependent antioxidant enzyme)

Other tests:
Gut Permeability
Increased

Haematology and Biochemistry
Enclosed for your kind attention

Ferritin
Enclosed for your kind attention

Thyroid Profile
Enclosed for your kind attention

I will address the nutritional deficiencies by using oral nutritional supplementation (sublingual for vitamin B12 – however, in view of the low status of Vitamin B12, you may wish to consider the administration of a course of Vitamin B12 injections).

The diet will be optimised, taking into account those foods which compromise the absorption of L-dopa medication.

Diet and supplements will be recommended for restoration of the integrity of the gut mucosa.

Bowel function will be optimised (Mrs Jay has a tendency to constipation).

I shall inform you of progress.

Thank you for your attention and assuring you of my co-operation in the best interests of Mrs Jay.

Yours sincerely

Lucille Leader Dip ION MBANT
Nutritional Therapist

Encl.

Medical Response!
The GP administered a 6 week course of vitamin B12 injections.

Different Scenarios Requiring Communication with the GP

Nutritional Therapist requesting Drug Review because of Side Effects

Lucille Leader Dip ION MBANT
Nutritional Therapist

Highgate Hospital
View Road
London N6 4DJ

Tel: 020 84454550
Fax: 020 84464504
Email: denor@dial.pipex.com

8th January 2009

Dr K Smith
The Gell Surgery
3 Hill Crescent
London N5 2JL

Dear Dr Smith

Re: Geoffrey Tom   **DOB: 01/11/1939, 53a Long Lane, Stamford, KT3 4AQ**

Mrs Tom has telephoned me in great distress because her husband is experiencing hallucinations since the commencement of the pharmaceutical Ropinerole. This was prescribed recently by his neurologist, Dr Tom Highfield. She feels that his paranoid behaviour is undermining her health – as you are aware, she is suffering from cancer.

I have advised Mr and Mrs Tom to make an appointment with you to review his drug regime.

Thank you for your kind attention to this urgent matter.

Yours sincerely

Lucille Leader Dip ION MBANT
Nutritional Therapist

> ## Medical Response!
> *The patient was referrred back to his neurologist who changed the medication.*

Notes:

Different Scenarios Requiring Communication with the GP

Nutritional Therapist's request for a "trial" of Drug Change in order to facilitate Dietary Flexibility

Lucille Leader Dip ION MBANT
Nutritional Therapist

Highgate Hospital
View Road
London N6 4DJ

Tel: 020 84454550
Fax: 020 84464504
Email: denor@dial.pipex.com

8th January 2009

Dr K Smith
The Gell Surgery
3 Hill Crescent
London N5 2JL

Dear Dr Smith

Re: Geoffrey Tom   DOB: 01/11/1939, 53a Long Lane, Stamford, KT3 4AQ

In monitoring drug-nutrient interactions, I have noted that Mr Tom's L-dopa medication (*Madopar* 100mg/25mg - capsule) takes one hour to "kick-in".

As this compromises dietary flexibility, would you consider prescribing a week's trial of L-dopa medication in the form of *Madopar* 100mg/25mg - Dispersible? The dispersible formula is more rapidly absorbed.

Thank you for your kind consideration of this request.

Yours sincerely

Lucille Leader Dip ION MBANT
Nutritional Therapist

see over for Medical Response ➡

Medical Response!
The GP gave the patient 10 days worth of Madopar Dispersible and the result was that it was indeed better absorbed...within 30 minutes.

This gave relief of symptoms within half the time and allowed for better dietary flexibility (this drug, which contains L-dopa, interacts with the large neutral amino acids in the diet and therefore needs to be administered away from food).

Different Scenarios Requiring Communication with the GP

Nutritional Therapist's Request for Referral to Speech Therapist

Lucille Leader Dip ION MBANT
Nutritional Therapist

Highgate Hospital
View Road
London N6 4DJ

Tel: 020 84454550
Fax: 020 84464504
Email: denor@dial.pipex.com

8th January 2009

Dr K Smith
The Gell Surgery
3 Hill Crescent
London N5 2JL

Dear Dr Smith

Re: Sarah Jones DOB: 14/01/1945, 136 Highcroft, Glasgow, G4 8FG

As you know, Mrs Jones attends our clinic for nutritional management. She was diagnosed with Multiple Sclerosis in March 2000.

Ms Jones has recently started experiencing dysphagia as well as problems with speech projection. As such, I have asked her to consult you about referral to a neuro speech therapist.

I shall closely monitor progress as she may well need referral, in the future, for tube feeding.

Thank you for your attention and assuring you of my co-operation in the best interests of Mrs Jones.

Yours sincerely

Lucille Leader
Nutritional Therapist Dip ION MBANT

see over for Medical Response ➡

Medical Response!
The patient was referred to a speech therapist who was later able to assess that swallowing was unsafe. She therefore recommended tube feeding rather than oral nutrition (in the interests of safety) and the patient went on to hospital nutritional management).

Different Scenarios Requiring Communication with the GP

Nutritional Therapist's Request for Assessment of Intestinal Pathology

Lucille Leader Dip ION MBANT
Nutritional Therapist

Highgate Hospital
View Road
London N6 4DJ

Tel: 020 84454550
Fax: 020 84464504
Email: denor@dial.pipex.com

8th January 2009

Dr K Smith
The Gell Surgery
3 Hill Crescent
London N5 2JL

Dear Dr Smith

Re: Jane Dee DOB 2/02/1948, 136 Highstone Rd, London L5 9DJ

As you know, Ms Dee attends my clinic for nutritional management. She was diagnosed with Parkinson's Disease in January 2000.

At her recent consultation with me she reported that she was passing blood and mucus in the stool. Additionally, an unusual dark and itchy lesion has recently appeared on her right hand. I have asked her to consult you urgently for your kind assessment.

Thank you for your attention and assuring you of my co-operation in the best interests of Ms Dee.

Yours sincerely

Lucille Leader Dip ION MBANT
Nutritional Therapist

see over for Medical Response ➡

Medical Response!
The GP telephoned the patient to come in urgently for consultation. She was referred for two specialist assessments.

A gastroenterologist established that she was suffering from ulcerative colitis. Her skin lesion is being monitored regularly by a dermatologist.

Different Scenarios Requiring Communication with the GP

Nutritional Therapist's Alert to the GP about Urgent Medical Problems

Lucille Leader Dip ION MBANT
Nutritional Therapist

Highgate Hospital
View Road
London N6 4DJ

Tel: 020 84454550
Fax: 020 84464504
Email: denor@dial.pipex.com

8th January 2009

Dr P Patel
3 Adcock Lane
Leeds
M3 5EP

Dear Dr Patel

Re: Ron Sanger: DOB: 1/9/1945, The Kenns, Oak Road, Leeds, M3 5HT

Thank you for your kind referral of Mr Sanger for nutritional assessment and recommendation. He presented with hypertension controlled by *Amlodipine*. He is hypothyroid, takes "*Armour*" thyroid and suffers from "restless legs".

I have asked Mr Sanger to see you as soon as possible for your kind assessment of the following problems:

a) I enclose results of tests (haematology, ferritin and biochemistry) organised by me. The extremely low status of haemoglobin, iron saturation and ferritin is of grave concern.

b) Oedema (feet and ankles). He easily becomes breathless and is unable to exercise or walk any distance.

c) Biochemical tests at Biolab Medical Unit in London demonstrated the following nutritional deficiencies: Vitamin B12, folate, zinc and magnesium.

continued over ➡

I shall address the deficiencies using sublingual nutrients where possible. However, you may wish to consider vitamin B12 injections in view of the low haematinic status.

Assuring you of my co-operation in the best interests of Mr Sanger.

Yours sincerely

Lucille Leader Dip ION MBANT
Nutritional Therapist

> ### *Medical Response!*
> *This patient was referred for blood transfusion the same day that the GP received this letter (which was sent by urgent fax). He was found to be bleeding in the intestinal tract and suffering from pernicious anaemia.*
>
> *He was also referred to a cardiologist who treated him for heart failure.*

Different Scenarios Requiring Communication with the GP

Nutritional Therapist Relinquishing Responsibility for Nutritional Care due to Unexplained Weight-loss in a Patient

Lucille Leader Dip ION MBANT
Nutritional Therapist

Highgate Hospital
View Road
London N6 4DJ

Tel: 020 84454550
Fax: 020 84464504
Email: denor@dial.pipex.com

8th January 2009

Dr P Patel
3 Adcock Lane
Leeds
M3 5EP

Dear Dr Patel

Re: Helen Bunker, DOB: 23/7/43, 31 New St, Ipswich IP8 1AU

Mrs Bunker has lost a stone in weight over the past month. Despite adequate calorie intake together with special supplementation (designer protein Allergy Research: "IMUPlus", which is appropriate for cancer patients), she has nevertheless continued to lose weight. I feel that this significant weight loss is now outside my brief as a Nutritional Therapist.

I have asked Mrs Bunker to make an urgent appointment with you for your further assessment and recommendation.

Thank you for your kind attention.

Yours sincerely

Lucille Leader Dip ION MBANT
Nutritional Therapist

see over for Medical Response ➡

Medical Response!

On receiving this letter by urgent fax, the GP telephoned the patient to come in immediately for consultation. Mrs Bunker was diagnosed with breast cancer some years back but had been in remission when she came for nutritional assessment and recommendation.

The GP referred her for tests and she appeared to be suffering from malignancy once again. Her care was therefore taken over by an oncology team.

Nonetheless, I wrote to the GP and recommended a medical physician who works with nutrition as adjuvant care for oncology patients. Some years later, this patient is still functioning well, albeit under medical nutritional care.

Different Scenarios Requiring Communication with the GP

Nutritional Therapist's Alert about a Patient possibly "at risk"

Lucille Leader Dip ION MBANT
Nutritional Therapist

Highgate Hospital
View Road
London N6 4DJ

Tel: 020 84454550
Fax: 020 84464504
Email: denor@dial.pipex.com

8th January 2009

Dr M Smythe
TheWinston Surgery
5 Hocroft Lane
London N12 5 NL

Dear Dr Smythe

Re: Walter Rose, DOB 12.01.1948, 12 Lee St, West Finchley, N12 6AB
    Tel: 07743 122766

I have spoken to our mutual patient, Mr Rose, this morning. He appeared to be very depressed and agitated.

In view of his medical history, I am concerned that he may be "at risk". I am therefore sending you this letter by fax for your urgent attention and kind assessment of the situation.

Assuring you of my co-operation with you at all times in the best and safe interests of Mr Rose.

Yours sincerely

Lucille Leader Dip ION MBANT
Nutritional Therapist

see over for Medical Response ➡

Duty of Care, Ethics, Client/Patient Confidentiality

The Nutritional Therapist has a duty of care to the client/patient. Patient confidentially is vital. However, should the therapist feel that the client/patient could pose a danger to him/herself or others, it is prudent to alert the GP. If there is any doubt or if there are ethical problems, the professional body of the therapist should be contacted for guidance.

When the Oral Route Fails

Part 1: Enteral Feeding (through the gut)

Elemental Feeding

Elemental feeds consist of pre-digested fluids which contain macro and micro nutrients in a healthy balance (all the elements).

Elemental feeding can be prescribed for oral and tube administration.
The amount of feeding is calculated by the number of calories needed for the size of the patient.

The product chosen depends on patients' biochemical individuality and dietary/nutrient requirements.
An example is *Peptamen* (Nestlé).

Elemental drinks can be added to a normal oral diet between meals, if the patient is needing extra nutritional support.

However, these specialised liquid formulae are designed to replace solid food completely under specific conditions.

These are:
- patients are unable to swallow
- patients have acute inflammatory bowel disease
- patients have post surgical problems of digestion and absorption
- patients suffer from malabsorption
- patients have intestinal pathology which prevents adequate digestion and absorption of macro and micro-nutrients

Notes:

When the Oral Route Fails

Elemental *Oral* Feeding

Patients can take the elemental liquid feed orally if swallowing is not a problem.

Elemental *Tube* Feeding

Tube feeding is recommended when patients cannot swallow or have difficulty in doing so.

Methods of Introduction

Specialised elemental formulae are passed from a 'food pack' through a tube into the body. There are two methods

- the tube is inserted through the nose, extending down to the stomach (nasogastric tube)

or alternatively

- the tube is inserted surgically directly into the duodenum (duodenal tube).

Important Note

Duodenal feeding is (anecdotally) less traumatic for patients.

Only when possible and if safe: it is important for patients with nasogastric and duodenal tubes to try to swallow a little water or other appropriate clear liquid over the day in order to reduce atrophy that may occur in the oesophagus and intestinal tract. This must be under the strict supervision of the attending medical team.

Notes:

When the Oral Route Fails

Nutritional Therapist's Request for Elemental Feeding

Lucille Leader Dip ION MBANT
Nutritional Therapist

Highgate Hospital
View Road
London N6 4DJ

Tel: 020 84454550
Fax: 020 84464504
Email: denor@dial.pipex.com

8th January 2009

Dr P Patel
3 Adcock Lane
Leeds
M3 5EP

Dear Dr Patel

Re: Jacqueline Baker, DOB: 14/01/1945, 136 Highcroft Gardens, Glasgow G42 K34

As you know, Mrs Baker attends my clinic for nutritional management. She was diagnosed with Crohn's Disease in March 2000.

Mrs Baker is experiencing a flare-up of her condition. As such, it would be greatly appreciated if you could prescribe 2 weeks supply of an elemental feed which she will be able to take orally, to replace solid food.

Research and clinical experience demonstrate that 'bowel rest' during an inflammatory episode often ameliorates patient discomfort and speeds remission. The NHS formulation which is appropriate for Crohn's Disease is *Peptamen* manufactured by Nestlé. This does not contain casein or gluten and is a comprehensive poly-peptide based formula. It has an excellent track record.

I recommend the following prescription:
Nestlé: *Peptamen* 200ml (200 kcal), vanilla flavour
       8 cups daily (providing 1600 calories)

Thank you for your kind attention and assuring you of my continuing co-operation in the best interests of Mrs Baker.

Yours sincerely

Lucille Leader Dip ION MBANT
Nutritional Therapist

see over for Medical Response ➡

Medical Response!
The GP prescribed the requested Peptamen to replace solid food for two weeks. The patient's acute inflammatory period settled down and she went into remission.

When the Oral Route Fails

Nutritional Therapist Relinquishing Responsibility

Lucille Leader Dip ION MBANT
Nutritional Therapist

Highgate Hospital	Tel: 020 84454550
View Road	Fax: 020 84464504
London N6 4DJ	Email: denor@dial.pipex.com

8th January 2009

Dr P Patel
3 Adcock Lane
Leeds
M3 5EP

Dear Dr Patel

Re: Claire Harris, DOB: 01/11/1935, 3a Long Lane, Stamford, KT3 4AQ

Mrs Harris suffers from Multiple Sclerosis diagnosed in March 1994. Due to increased dysphagia, Mrs Harris is unable to eat sufficiently to sustain health.

I have asked her to consult you urgently for assessment and consideration of referral for tube feeding. I am unable to take responsibility for her nutritional management whilst she is in this condition.

Thank you for your kind co-operation.

Yours sincerely

Lucille Leader Dip ION MBANT
Nutritional Therapist

Medical Response!
The GP referred the patient for tube feeding. She gained and maintained weight under the management of a hospital dietician. After some weeks, after going into remission, she was able to tolerate normal oral nutrition again .

Notes:

When the Oral Route Fails

Part 2: Parenteral Nutrition (outside the gut)

Intravenous Total Parenteral Nutrition (TPN)

When it is medically necessary to completely exclude the gastro-intestinal tract, patients receive their total nutrition intravenously. This method is known as - Total Parenteral Nutrition (TPN).

This complete feed, containing protein, fat, carbohydrate, vitamins and minerals is ideally administered via a central vein because peripheral veins may be easily irritated.

It is a stressful experience for patients. However, this technique saves lives when there is no alternative nutritional route.

Parenteral Administration of Individual Nutrients

The nutritional therapist can report failure of absorption of nutrients to the GP - despite oral therapeutic administration over a reasonable period.

Some deficiencies of nutrients which are unable to be corrected orally, are able to be administered intravenously (IV) or intra-muscularly (IM).

These include:

- Vitamins
- Minerals
- Glutathione

Notes:

When the Oral Route Fails

Nutritional Therapist Reporting Malabsorption of Nutrients

Lucille Leader Dip ION MBANT
Nutritional Therapist

Highgate Hospital
View Road
London N6 4DJ

Tel: 020 84454550
Fax: 020 84464504
Email: denor@dial.pipex.com

8th January 2009

Dr P Patel
3 Adcock Lane
Leeds
M3 5EP

Dear Dr Patel

Re: Mrs Elaine Tripp, DOB: 03/10/1940, 3a Libby Street, Stamford, LA2 4DB

As you know, Mrs Tripp attends my clinic for nutritional management. She suffers from Diverticulitis diagnosed in June 2000. Despite the administration of therapeutic doses of Vitamin B12 (sublingually) for this deficiency demonstrated in October 2008, her cellular status remains low (see the enclosed laboratory test results).

I have asked her to consult you for assessment and consideration of a course of injections to up-regulate this condition.

Thank you for your kind consideration of the above report.

Assuring you of my cooperation at all times in the best interests of Mrs Tripp.

Yours sincerely

Lucille Leader Dip ION MBANT
Nutritional Therapist

Medical Response!
The GP administered a course of vitamin B12 injections.

Notes:

Peri-Surgical Nutrition

Nutritional Management to Enhance Recovery from Surgery and Anaesthesia

Patients will be on different individual diets according to their pathologies. The Nutritional Therapist should ensure continuity at the hospital before the patient is admitted either by communication with the resident Dietician, Sister-in-Charge of the ward or with the Surgeon or Anaesthetist.

Undergoing Anaesthesia
by Dr Geoffrey Leader MB ChB FRCA and Lucille Leader Dip ION MBANT

Preoperatively

1. Two weeks before surgery (if time permits) ensure that patients cease taking nutrients which affect the clotting potential of the blood. These include vitamin C, vitamin E, Omega 6 (GLA) and Omega 3 (EPA).
2. There are also medicinal herbs which thin the blood. These should also be omitted. It is important to check the properties of nutrients and herbs and their interactions with drugs.
3. Patients should be advised to discuss their drug regimes with the surgeon /anaesthetist well before the surgery, time permitting.
4. Ensure that patients have good bowel function before surgery. If constipation is a problem, the following can be helpful, taken at *different intervals* over the day:
    a. Presoaked prunes and figs
    b. Adequate fluid
    c. *Caricol* (Nutri Ltd/Solgar)
    d. For five days prior to surgery red meat should be avoided. This requires a great deal of digestion and has a longer transit time through the gut than other protein sources.
    e. Alcohol should be avoided
    f. Caffeine - containing food and drinks should be reduced (tea, coffee, chocolate)

Notes:

5. Contemporary anaesthetic considerations include maintaining blood sugar levels and fluid prior to surgery. *Clear* fluids will have passed out of the stomach well before actual surgery[1, 2] if taken two to three hours before the event and therefore do not pose any risk during induction of anaesthesia[3].

Two to three hours before surgery a drink (150ml) can be taken which contains long chain glucose polymers such as *Ultra Fuel* (Twinlab) – 75ml of *Ultra Fuel* topped up with 75ml of still mineral or purified water.

If this is not available, a similar amount of dilute clear apple juice may be imbibed. The timing of taking this, or any clear fluid, should be confirmed with the attending anaesthestist before the date of surgery.

Post Surgery

After surgery, it is most suitable to replace the first meal with a polypeptide-based elemental liquid feed such as *Peptamen* (Nestlé). Being more easily and quickly absorbed than solid food, it is therefore more appropriate after surgery as digestion is not optimal at this time.

Administration of vitamins C and E, Essential Fatty Acids - Omega 6 and Omega 3, or any nutrients and medicinal herbs which affect platelet aggregation, should only be resumed after wound-healing has commenced.

Regulation of bowel function after surgery may pose a problem. This can be associated with analgesics. If constipation is unrelieved, guidance and permission for recommendations must always be obtained from the medical team.

Dopaminergic drugs (in Parkinson's disease) can be taken with a very small sip of water prior to surgery and post-operatively. However this must be authorised by the attendant anaesthetist. A Parkinson's Disease patient should arrange consultation with the anaesthetist before the day of surgery.

Notes:

Post-operatively (After Hospital Discharge)

Nutrients may be indicated for the restoration of the integrity of the gut mucosa, support of the effects of oxidative stress[4] and liver function.

These aspects should only be addressed after wound healing has commenced and the patient has been discharged. *A note to this effect should be sent to the GP.*

The concept of enhancing detoxification is an important one for general anaesthesia and particularly in Parkinson's Disease patients. However, in neurological cases[5, 6, 7,] it is important for the nutritional therapist not to indulge in dynamic detoxification protocols as the liver, however well supported, may not cope. Resuming a careful diet is the more prudent[8.]

Notes:

Nutritional Therapist Requesting Post Surgical Nutritional Prescription

Lucille Leader Dip ION MBANT
Nutritional Therapist

Highgate Hospital
View Road
London N6 4DJ

Tel: 020 84454550
Fax: 020 84464504
Email: denor@dial.pipex.com

3rd November 2007

Mr Colin Deed
Consultant Gynaecologist
28 Harley Street
London
W1 2GH

Dear Mr Deed

RE: Anne Golden, DOB 23/04/1955, 27 Grange Grove, Edgware, WR4 2YT

Would you kindly consider prescribing the following elemental liquid feed for Mrs Golden for post surgical nutritional administration? She will be undergoing hysterectomy. As you know, she suffers from The Irritable Bowel Syndrome (IBS) and a pre-digested liquid feed would be helpful for her.

Nestlé: *Peptamen* 200ml (200 kcals), vanilla flavour
　　　12 cups to be ordered

Directions for oral feeding:

Day 1: (6 – 8 cups). One 200ml cup to be taken at two-hourly intervals. This may be diluted (100ml *Peptamen* with 100ml still mineral water) if too rich for the patient immediately postoperatively.

Days 2, 3 and 4: One 200ml cup in place of the evening meal.

Thank you for your kind attention and assistance in the best interests of Mrs Golden.

Yours sincerely

Lucille Leader
Nutritional Therapist

Notes:

When would it be prudent to inform the General Practitioner that you are unable to maintain responsibility for Nutritional Care?

- When clients/patients are incapable of reliably sorting out an essential drug and/or nutritional regime.
- When clients/patients are unable to care adequately and safely for themselves.
- When clients/patients are not completely compliant – for example, a diabetic who does not monitor glucose levels regularly and does not keep strictly to specific nutritional recommendations.
- When there is infection that is not being treated by the GP/Medical Specialist.
- When there is inflammation that is not being treated by the GP/Medical Specialist.
- When there is pathology that is not being treated by the GP/Medical Specialist.
- When there are psychological and psychotic disorders that are not being treated by the GP/Psychiatrist/Psychologist.
- When there is dysphagia and/or chewing problems preventing safe swallowing.
- When there is unexplained weight loss/gain.
- Other conditions which are beyond the remit or training of the Nutritional Therapist.
- When the client/patient declines further nutritional therapy.

To summarise:
There are situations or conditions which can compromise the effectiveness of your nutritional recommendations due to circumstances beyond your control or beyond your remit and training as a clinical nutritionist/nutritional therapist. In the best and safe interests of the client/patient, it is advisable to inform the GP, as well as any other medical specialist involved with the case, that you are unable to take responsibility for nutritional care.

There could be legal implications should negative outcome be attributed to inappropriate nutritional management.

Notes:

References

1. Erskine L, Hunt JN: 1981: The gastric emptying of small volumes given in quick succession: J Physiol: 313: pps. 334-35

2. Brener W, Hendrix TR, McHugh R: 1983: Regulation of the gastric emptying of glucose: Gastroenterology: 85: pps. 76-82

3. Connolly J, Cunningham A: 2000: European Journal of Anaesthesiology: Vol. 17: Issue 4: pps. 219-220: Preoperative fasting and administration of regular administration of regular medications in adult patients presenting for elective surgery. Has new evidence changed clinical practice?

4. Beutler E: 1989: Nutritional and Metabolic Aspects of Glutathione: Annual Review of Nutrition Vol 9: pps. 287-302

5. C M Tanner: 1991: Abnormal Liver Enzyme-mediated Metabolism in Parkinson's Disease - A Second Look: Neurology 41: (5 suppl 2): pps. 89-92

6. Williams S, Sturman A, Steventon G, Waring R: 1991: Metabolic Biomarkers of Parkinson's Disease: Acta Neurologica Scandinavica: Supplementum 136: pps. 19-23

7. Liver Enzyme Abnormalities in Parkinson's Disease: 1991: Geriatrics 46 Suppl 1: pps. 60-63

8. Anderson KE, Kappas: 1991: A Dietary Regulation of Cytochrome P450: Annual Review of Nutrition Vol. 11: pps. 141-67